HYPOGLYCEMIA

What It Is, What It Isn't, and How to Fix the Root Problem

⟳ Matt Stone

A proud presentation of:

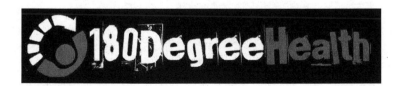

May 2014
Copyright © 2014 Archangel Ink

Published by Archangel Ink
ISBN: 1500209449
ISBN-13: 978-1500209445

DISCLAIMER

The material provided here is for educational and informational purposes only and is not intended as medical advice. The information contained in this book should not be used to diagnose or treat any illness, metabolic disorder, disease, or health problem. If you have developed a serious illness of some kind, the complexities of dealing with that disorder are best handled by your physician or other professional health care provider, whom you should also consult with before beginning any nutrition or exercise program. Use of the programs, advice, and other information contained in this book is at the sole choice and risk of the reader.

Table of Contents

Introduction

Hi I'm Matt Stone and I'm annoyed. For me personally, nothing on the face of the planet is more annoying than the improper use of the English language. Sure, I'm no stranger to an occasional grammatical error. I'm certain there will be at least a few errors in the pages ahead. But calling that shaky feeling some people get after meals or when they've gone too long without food "hypoglycemia" is just ridiculous.

It ranks up there with calling ice cream "carbs" (a food that is typically 62% *not* carbohydrate), or calling lard "saturated fat" when it is mostly unsaturated fat. Nowumsayinhereman?

Okay, maybe that's not my biggest annoyance. I did break a laptop once.

Sorry honey. You have to admit though, the replacement laptop is much better.

Anger management issues aside, the word "hypoglycemia" means: low…sugar…blood. How many people actually suffer from their blood sugar being low? Almost no one. It's extremely rare. That's why many doctors snicker when they hear "hypoglycemia." They think the condition basically doesn't even exist except in very rare cases or amongst diabetics who've accidentally taken too much insulin. And you know what? This is one of the few times that your poorly-educated doctor is absolutely right.

Way to go doc. But I still snicker when I hear the word "doctor." Please don't get even cockier than you already are because when it comes to hypoglycemia you're still a fool…

Despite the factual accuracy of the medical world's stance on hypoglycemia, they often absurdly do not acknowledge that something is going on. Sadly, doctors are more likely to diagnose you with hypochondria than hypoglycemia. The best mainstream term that has been created to describe this obnoxious, non-hypoglycemic, real-and-not-imagined condition of feeling shaky, irritable, anxious, dizzy, fatigued, disoriented, etc. at various points throughout the day is "Idiopathic Postprandial Syndrome." Just because this term is out there doesn't mean your doctor has heard of it either. He or she probably hasn't.

Idiopathic means that they don't know what the hell is going on, which is both idiotic and pathetic. Idiopathetic is where I was headed with that. The condition isn't all that mysterious in cause or cure. It involves many factors such as metabolic rate, adrenal hormones, electrolyte balances, and glucose metabolism. In many cases it can be easily improved. In other cases that I haven't been able to crack, I still maintain faith that there is a solution out there—a solution that can be obtained with some decent guidance.

So I write this short book to delve into the topic of Hypoglycemia with a mix of experience, research, speculation, anecdote, and observation by past clinicians with an interest in this condition. From that is birthed some guidance on how you, an individual who may suffer from this obnoxious affliction to some degree, can go about improving this problem through your own self-experimentation.

Without further ado let's dive straight in to this interesting topic…

The Hypoglycemia Myth

Once upon a time I referred to "hypoglycemia" casually just like everybody else. One time that was particularly memorable was in reference to my girlfriend, who has suffered from epilepsy since age seven.

I noticed some interesting things in my girlfriend early on in our relationship. For example, when her behavior changed to suggest that she was becoming "seizure-ish," a spoonful of sugar in her mouth would immediately revive her. Crackers and other snacks worked great if she was still fully coherent but starting to feel "shaky."

Also, I noticed that one of the biggest risks in terms of triggering a seizure was eating a big meal. While eating looked like a problem on the surface, the more she didn't eat, the more likely she was to have a seizure when she did eat. Calling it a precarious situation is an understatement. She was in a rough place when I met her. We'll talk about some of those phenomena later. Don't worry; she's in a much better place now.

I bring this up because a good friend of hers is a paramedic. Her paramedic friend knew she was having seizure trouble and started doling out obnoxious and downright dangerous advice—encouraging her to start drinking a lot of water for example, which, for reasons we'll delve into later, is a terrible idea.

In one of those new-fashioned aggressive online debates with a perfect stranger, I called her friend on this poor health advice, pointed out some studies showing that water can actually cause seizures, and generally patronized the heck out of her with a very likeable tone that suggested, "I'm Matt F$#%ing Stone. Who the hell are you?"

Always keepin' it classy! "Computer screen bravado" I think they call that, which is actually a pretty interesting new form of human behavior that I'm a big fan of. That's why I spend so much time communicating with people online. On the internet, people are actually honest and don't waste time with small talk and spineless pleasantries!

During this communication with the paramedic, I mentioned something about "hypoglycemia" being the primary trigger of my girlfriend's seizures and got a good laugh out of her. She was like, "Hypoglycemia? Are you kidding me? Do you really think when we test the blood sugar of someone who just had a seizure in the back of an ambulance that it's low? Let me tell you, it's never low. It's always high! You're wrong you dumb @#$&*%@#%(@#%!!!"

I quickly explained that this phenomenon cannot be detected in the blood, that I shouldn't have called it "hypoglycemia," and that when blood sugar falls it's not detectable because the adrenal glands turn on to raise blood sugar. In one of these stressful events (seizure) the outpouring of adrenaline actually makes blood sugar surge. That was all true, but it was clear that I had opened the door for harsh criticism. There was a chink in my armor. I had to stop using the H word, because using the H word, which means low blood sugar, and then explaining how blood sugar becomes elevated from "hypoglycemia" just makes no sense, and leaves me looking like the absolute last thing I want to look like—a pseudoscientific quack guru moron (PQGM).

So let's talk about this myth known as "hypoglycemia."

I laid out a pretty good synopsis of hypoglycemia already. Something sets off a stress reaction in the body and the adrenal glands switch on. Accompanying this surge in adrenal

hormones—let's just call them "glucocorticoids"—
are some fairly reliable physical and mental changes.
Pulse rate rises. When severe it feels like heart
palpitations. Feelings of anxiety or aggression can
kick in, as expected when the "fight or flight"
hormones rise. Shakiness, even trembling can occur
if severe. Lightheadedness is common as are
headaches and sometimes migraines and seizures if
more severe. Icy cold fingers and toes as the blood
vessels in the extremities close up are frequently
noted. A sudden, strong urge to urinate or frequent
urination often occurs—like proverbially "peeing
your pants" when you get really scared (causing
those glucocorticoids to surge).

And, these "gluco" (as in glucose) –corticoids
raise blood sugar to deliver emergency fuel to the
body's cells. They dump free fatty acids into the
bloodstream as well, which can further raise blood
sugar as free fatty acids interfere with glucose
uptake.

The problem is that there are many triggers of
this phenomenon. Classical idiopathic postprandial
syndrome, where eating is the primary trigger of this
phenomenon is the primary focus of this book, but
it would be a disservice not to look from a broader
perspective.

So I don't even think we should limit
ourselves to the definition of idiopathic
postprandial syndrome, as episodes like this are just

as likely to occur in the fasted state at 4am as they are right after a meal. I don't know what else to do other than craft a new name. In the past I've called them "adrenaline surges" or something similar, but I fear even that as there are probably other hormones involved besides adrenaline.

Can we be safe and call this problem "adrenergic syndrome" and remove the word "postprandial" from it altogether? Adrenergic as in adrenal gland activity? Okay good. I hope so.

The first big question then… What causes adrenergic syndrome?

Cause of Adrenergic Syndrome

Oh boy, here we go. Not only have we identified a constellation of symptoms, we've crafted ourselves a new disease. Now we're already talking about the cause of this syndrome. Some PQGM stuff going on right here for sure. Oh well, we'll ignore the naysayers who want to bash this book and my work. They'll find a way to do that no matter what. If you suffer from this problem to some degree though, I know you're all ears. And I really do have some helpful information to share with you (that isn't the standard "eat protein, small meals, and avoid carbs"), or I wouldn't be writing this book (which I am writing on Christmas at the very moment I typed that last sentence—not sure exactly what that's supposed to mean, but I do have quite a bit of "passion" for this kinda thing or I'd be drunk off eggnog right now or whatever it is that normal people do).

What is the cause of adrenergic syndrome? That's a tough question. Here are some fragments of information that I know for sure from my years of experience, observation, and study:

1. Lowering your metabolic rate makes it worse in almost a linear fashion, meaning that the problem happens more frequently and the symptoms become increasingly severe.

2. Reduced metabolic rate is already established as a causative factor if one is to consider the work of Broda Barnes, who used thyroid medication to raise metabolic rate and allegedly fix the condition.

3. The more stressed out you are, the more likely you are to experience the postprandial version. The most common forms of stress are being very busy, emotional events, not getting very good sleep, and going too many hours without food. These types of stressors frequently set a person up for an even bigger crash landing when they finally do eat.

4. Consuming too many fluids in proportion to calories, carbohydrates, and salt can trigger the syndrome in susceptible individuals.

5. Potassium seems to make it worse, while sodium seems to make it better.

6. The most common times to experience the syndrome is roughly 2-4am and 9-11am. Experiencing it at other times of day is rare unless you skip breakfast. The postprandial version is most commonly experienced after breakfast, and some interesting dynamics between insulin and cortisol are discussed and referenced in an article written by Martin Berkhan entitled "Why Does Breakfast Make Me Hungry?"

7. 2-4am is when adrenaline is at its highest and body temperature (a marker of metabolic rate) is at its lowest, according to the extensive appendix on human circadian rhythms in the book Rhythms of Life.

8. Rapidly-absorbed carbohydrates paired with salt alleviates it most consistently (saltine crackers, let's say) when it's happening.

9. Frequent, pale or clear urination often accompanies it, or a strong sudden urge to urinate that comes seemingly out of nowhere but is very intense.

10.   It usually coincides with acute cold hands and feet and acute feelings of total body coldness, commonly experienced when the sympathetic nervous system (the stress side of the nervous system) becomes hyperactive.

11.   Food, particularly sugar, starch, and salt, which I've identified as the primary anti-adrenergic foods (the "Anti-Stress S's" I call them) —are helpful in an acute situation but are also excellent for preventing the condition and even eliminating it completely as part of a pro-metabolism, anti-stress dietary/lifestyle protocol. I developed what I call "rest and refeeding" strategies and noticed right away that they helped to improve or eliminate the tendency to have adrenergic surges. That discovery was the primary impetus for writing this book and sharing my insights.

12.   It's also common to experience the syndrome shortly after waking up from a nap.

When you put the above 12 items together it starts to paint a pretty vivid picture of what is going on in those with adrenergic syndrome and how to improve the condition.

By the way, please don't start thinking in absolutes now that we have some items on a list. I fear what would happen if, for example, I say that eating a low-carb diet causes this condition. Based on many individual cases that I've dealt with, I would say that it's very common to develop adrenergic syndrome from prolonged carbohydrate restriction. However, there are also many people who used to have the condition, but now they no longer suffer from it after switching to a low-carb diet. So we shouldn't think of causes in that sense. Instead, think of *physiology*. Being in a particular physiological state causes the condition, and for any particular individual, the cause of getting into that susceptible state can be anything under the sun.

If that's confusing, let me put it this way…

There is a vegan, a low-carber, a Paleo eater, someone who just lost a loved one, a baby drinking poor-quality milk, a competitive athlete, a person drinking way too much water, a gamer, someone with an eating disorder, and a regular Joe couch potato all suffering from this condition right now. And all of their daily habits, diets, and health practices have contributed to their problem. There isn't a single cause in that sense. Anything can cause it. The trick is identifying the physiological state that has resulted and following some reasonable strategies to climb out of that state.

Put even more simply, there are many paths leading to the same destination. And if you find yourself suffering from adrenergic syndrome, you probably need to do something different than what you are doing right now.

If there is any way to unify all these causes, it would be to say that...

Anything causing a rise in stress hormones and a drop in metabolic rate makes the emergence of the condition more likely. Where it exists already, a drop in metabolic rate and a rise in glucocorticoids is likely to make it worse.

Now that we've laid a little foundation, let's examine an interesting facet of adrenergic syndrome that provides more clues as to what's really going on—the *time of day* when people are most likely to experience acute episodes.

Circadian Rhythms: Clues for Approaching the Problem

I t's 4am. For some strange reason you have awakened. You have a strong urge to pee. Your heart rate seems to be elevated. You may feel ravenous—so hungry it hurts. But it's a weird hunger that's different from what you typically experience. And, worst of all, you feel really alert. You've got a big day coming up and the last thing you want to be is tired and run down. You need to go back to sleep, but your mind races. You feel like you just had a cup of coffee and are wide awake.

There are many different manifestations of this pre-dawn phenomenon. The above is one that includes several generalizations. Other problems people may experience with the 2-4am wakeup is heart palpitations, extreme dry mouth/thirst, anxiety or a feeling of panic, extreme coldness or sweating, and other symptoms. Interestingly, many people seem to go off like this as if an alarm clock were set to it. People say things to me like:

"3:17am every day. It's so weird."

That's because this adrenergic pulse or "adrenaline surge" is regulated by our internal clock—the Circadian Rhythms, which are incredibly precise. Everyone has a time of day that is his or her physiological low point. In a normal person, this commonly falls between 2-4am. At this time, adrenaline reaches its peak. It does this, I believe, because metabolism is at its lowest level. The metabolic rate is in charge of stimulating cells to generate energy. As it falls and energy becomes scarce, adrenaline surges as a form of backup, or, a secondary energy. In other words, a lack of energy is stressful and causes a rise in adrenaline to compensate for this emergency state.

Okay, maybe that's being overly general, but for the purposes of getting practical benefits, that's a good working understanding of this metabolism-adrenaline seesaw.

What increases adrenaline lowers true metabolic energy. What increases metabolic energy tends to decrease adrenaline. That's why doing anything to decrease your metabolic rate can make the adrenergic surges start to occur with greater frequency and greater severity. Likewise, work that you do to increase your metabolic rate has a way of deactivating your sympathetic nervous system—decreasing the severity and frequency of your adrenergic surges.

If an improvement in metabolism lowers your adrenergic surges enough, you stop waking up when your adrenaline peaks during that 2-4am window. There are many types and many causes of sleep problems, but the metabolic enhancement program that I have written about in other books has had, as a side effect, a powerful ability to eliminate many people's sleep problems. Not in everyone of course. In fact, I find resolving a true case of severe insomnia to be one of the most difficult problems to solve.

So that's neat and all. Seems I was going somewhere with that. Um, oh yeah…

What I'm getting at with all this is that metabolism-stimulating, stress-suppressing dietary and lifestyle interventions are strongly indicated in anyone who has a tendency to feel these adrenergic spikes. We will get to a few basics in this book to be sure.

There is another interesting common time for people to have these adrenergic spikes though…

And that's the typical "Idiopathic Postprandial Syndrome" that occurs 1-2 hours after breakfast—usually between 9-11am. Although a person can crash at any time, this is without a doubt the most common time to experience it. This is presumably because stress hormones are higher and metabolism is lower in the morning than at any other time of day in a typical person. While adrenaline peaks earlier, cortisol peaks just after, and the higher cortisol goes, the bigger the postprandial insulin spike.

A half hour or so after a person wakes, cortisol really surges (in a typical person)—known as the "cortisol awakening response (CAR)." When a person eats food, protein and carbohydrates in particular, blood sugar rises and insulin is released to sweep that sugar out of the blood and into carbohydrate reserves in muscles and organs. The higher insulin goes after a meal, typically the faster blood sugar falls. Many believe that it is not true "hypoglycemia" that causes the adrenergic surge, but that a rapid descent in blood sugar levels can sound the glucocorticoid alarm. The glucocorticoids, if you remember, raise blood sugar—a defense against rapidly-falling blood sugar levels. This surge in glucocorticoids is probably responsible for the vast majority of the symptoms people experience with adrenergic syndrome.

If you think back to what I said about my girlfriend, this makes sense. Generally, the longer a person fasts, the bigger the rise in cortisol. The larger the rise in cortisol, the bigger the post-meal insulin spike, and the bigger the post-meal insulin spike, the more likely a person is to experience an adrenergic surge—even beyond the adrenal activity one might experience from fasting. The adrenergic surge was triggering seizure activity in my girlfriend. You don't have to know many epileptics to immediately recognize the stress-seizure connection.

Personally, I find nothing is more likely to trigger negative post-breakfast symptoms than a poor night's sleep. I think many people have gotten into the habit of eating and then paying attention to how their body responds to certain foods as if these foods are interacting with their bodies in a closed system with no other variables. When a person getting poor sleep eats a classic high-carbohydrate American-style breakfast (cereal, toast, juice, jam, oatmeal, fruit, smoothies, etc.), post-meal malaise is sure to strike. On the surface, many have made the tragic error of assuming that this type of breakfast "causes low blood sugar." In reality, one could easily argue that the vast majority of health problems seen in the modern world are caused by ever-decreasing amounts of sleep. Everyone blames certain foods, but in my experience everyone can change their body's reaction to most foods, often without any reliance on changes in diet.

To help you grasp this better, if someone came to me and said "eating carbs at breakfast makes me crash hard after," I would view this as a definite clue, not that carbs are bad for this person, but that there is something wrong with this person. The first question I would ask is "How many hours do you sleep per night?" And as you will soon read in another chapter, the person is more likely to be experiencing problems due to the water content in those carbohydrates, not the carbohydrates themselves.

Sleep loss is just one factor that can contribute to post-meal adrenergic syndrome. Any number of things can trigger an elevation in cortisol, and an elevation in cortisol is one of the most likely culprits in postprandial adrenergic syndrome.

So the clues we can gather from both the 2-4am wakeup and the common post-breakfast bomb are very simple and boil down to raising metabolism and lowering stress hormones. When you look at dietary and lifestyle interventions through this lens, a very different picture emerges than what has become standard health advice—from the mainstream, the fringes, or the fanatics. We'll get to that part for sure. Hold on though. First, a few important chapters—one for carbophobic "hypoglycemics" that are overly-infatuated with protein, another for those who experience extreme fatigue after meals and have wrongly dubbed this a "blood sugar crash," and another chapter to introduce an entirely different but very common cause of adrenergic syndrome that doesn't seem to be on anyone's radar screen…

High-Protein Diets

For ages the recommended diet for someone who suffers from apparent "hypoglycemia," which we now know should be called something more like adrenergic syndrome, is to eat often, and eat a lot of protein and not so many carbs—particularly simple sugars.

And this diet works pretty well. It gets the job done for the most part. What's the problem then? Well, I think there are many problems just as Broda Barnes did. In *Hope for Hypoglycemia* he writes…

"To date, when the symptoms of hypothyroidism are relieved, hypoglycemia, like the others, disappears. The diagnosis of hypothyroidism can be made from a careful history and physical examination better than it can from laboratory procedures. I routinely use the Basal Temperature test to confirm suspicions of hypothyroidism."

He goes on to write...

"It has been clearly established that a high protein diet lowers the metabolic rate, [therefore] symptoms of hypothyroidism will be aggravated… Hypoglycemia may be controlled on the high protein diet, but the other symptoms of thyroid deficiency which usually accompany hypoglycemia are aggravated."

Protein resurfaces again in Broda Barnes's *Hypothyroidism: The Unsuspecting Illness:*

"When the diet was changed so that it was low in fat but high in protein and with enough carbohydrate to prevent diarrhea, symptoms of hypothyroidism appeared. Cholesterol level in the blood became elevated and in order to keep it within normal range, four additional grains of thyroid daily were needed. Apparently, a diet high in protein requires additional thyroid for its metabolism."

I don't take the observations of the grand-high priest of all things metabolism very lightly. I can't agree wholeheartedly with everything the guy has ever written. Who could do that with anyone? But I've seen nothing but trouble with high-protein diets, with or without the restriction of carbohydrates. Protein, especially protein from meat, is very high in amino acids that are inflammatory and anti-metabolic, such as methionine, cysteine, and tryptophan. Very few have written much about the negative effects of these amino acids other than Ray Peat, but the evidence that amino acids like methionine or tryptophan in excess are toxic is pretty vast.

So, while eating a diet built primarily around meat and vegetables with perhaps a little starch is the typical recommendation to prevent "hypoglycemic" episodes, this dietary intervention does nothing to fix the root problem. In fact, if the root cause in adrenergic syndrome really is a reduced metabolic rate, and my experience with it strongly corroborates that possibility, then adopting a high-protein, low-carbohydrate diet could worsen the problem and exacerbate other hypothyroid symptoms precisely as Barnes claimed.

What I encourage you to do if you are a long-term sufferer from adrenergic syndrome is to think outside the box here a little bit. If you know that having a stack of pancakes covered with syrup and a glass of juice is going to cause a massive adrenergic event an hour or two later, that's merely a sign that something isn't working properly. Instead of strictly avoiding what seems like a trigger meal, all interventions should be judged on their ability to improve your tolerance for this trigger meal.

Just because that meal currently causes you great malaise doesn't mean that it is destined to stay that way forever. You can fix that. Most people can at least. You don't have to throw in the towel and retreat to a safe diet of meat and low-glycemic carbohydrates or whatever you've found to be a sure thing in avoiding this problem in the past. If someone can eat such a meal and maintain a healthy physical and mental state, odds are you can too with the right twists and tweaks.

Trust me. I know people who have gone from literally passing out unconscious from the rice and sugar in a sushi roll to obliterating a "hypoglycemic's" worst nightmare while feeling fine after the meal. Great actually.

So, suspend your trusted faith in what you've found to "work" in the past. If you still have to avoid certain carbohydrate-rich foods, or eat a hand-sized slab of chicken or fish with every baked potato to keep from feeling awful, you certainly haven't fixed the problem. You haven't fixed your hypoglycemia any more than someone avoiding peanuts has cured his or her peanut allergy. There is a great possibility that you can fix the problem altogether, not have to be bound by certain macronutrient ratios to keep from feeling psychotic, and clear up some metabolism-related conditions along with it.

Speaking from my own experience, when I first went on a more meat-based diet with lots of protein and very little carbohydrate, I felt incredible. Never before had I felt so emotionally stable. My energy levels were rock solid as well. It was heaven. I hadn't even realized that I had been on such an emotional rollercoaster prior. The positive changes

I felt after switching to a meat based diet made such a strong impression on me, that, you know, I started blogging and wrote a book about it. I was out to save the world from all those carbohydrates, you know?

Well, that was embarrassing. One of the first signs of trouble was a worsening of the rollercoaster ride when I ate any carbohydrates. Maybe I was a little moody before, but after a year or two on a low-carb diet, eating a single banana would have me breaking down and weeping for a whole day like I had a really bad case of dude PMS. And then the carbs made my teeth hurt. They made me gain weight. They made me break out with pimples. Hmmm. Eating carbs never did that to me before I started living la vida low carb.

Anyway, the high-protein, low-carb infatuation turned out to be a six-month honeymoon followed by feeling a lot worse than I felt before I started the diet. That was just a short list of problems I eventually encountered before waking up from my low-carb coma.

Now, times are good. I can eat almost anything and feel perfectly fine. No pimples, no tooth pain, no nothing. Just warm, normal, and steady.

Well, I feel good if I spend time outdoors, get some exercise, and don't stay up too late!

Okay, moving onward now to bigger and better things. I did think it was important to lay down a few mentions about the shortcomings of the standard "hypoglycemia" recommendations. They don't solve anything and may do you harm, especially when the cumulative mediocrity of such a diet catches up to you after years of trying to "control" your blood sugar problem. And, more importantly as we move forward—even if eating loads of carbohydrates makes you feel miserable right now, and odds are they will at the start, that is no excuse to retreat unless your adrenergic syndrome is severe enough to be life-threatening. Suicide, or even the thoughts of suicide deserves a special mention as it is probably the biggest risk for those who suffer from severe psychological malaise when their adrenal glands take them on a daily rollercoaster ride.

Postprandial Food Coma Syndrome

Many of you reading up to this point are wondering what all this talk of feeling aggressive, anxious, shaky, and cold is all about. From what you've been led to believe, a drop in blood sugar causes a drop in energy. You have been noticing feeling extremely tired, warm, and downright drowsy when eating the typical "hypoglycemia" triggers for years. You thought this was your blood sugar crashing. Probably not. It's also not necessarily a bad reflection on the particular foods that make you feel so sleepy and unfocused.

Feeling sleepy after eating is talked about in the peculiar place called the "alternative health realm of the internet" like it's a tumor or heart attack waiting to happen. Seriously, I hear crazy things about feeling sleepy after eating, the most common is that if you feel tired after eating something, then you must be "allergic" to that food. Come on man. This way of thinking lacks complete understanding of human physiology.

Do you really think a lion hops up after mowing down a half of a wildebeest and then goes for a voluntary jog because the meal was so energizing? I don't either. It's intuitive to feel calm, relaxed, warm, and drowsy after eating to fullness. It's normal to feel this way when blood sugar rises, not falls.

While glucocorticoids are the primary hormones that drive blood sugar up, insulin is the hormone that primarily drives blood sugar down. When you've just eaten, your blood sugar is going up, and the body wants to bring that blood sugar back to normal. The glucocorticoids generally shut down in proportion to the rise in insulin and blood sugar. While we obviously don't want blood sugar to go too high, and it won't if you are truly healthy no matter what you eat, it's simply normal physiology. It's certainly nothing to get too concerned about.

My perspectives on post-meal drowsiness was revealed in an April, 2013 article I wrote—one of the most heavily-viewed articles I've ever written…

There are three quick answers to the common question, 'Why am I sleepy after I eat?'

1. Because you're stressed.

2. Because you didn't sleep enough.

3. Because you ate enough.

Everyone in the health industry thinks that eating a meal should make you perk up and want to instantly break out into the Humpty Dance or other similar variant. Maybe throw in a high-intensity interval while you're at it. Just for kicks. If you do get sleepy after eating, your nutritionist or dietitian is ready to send you off to the lab for food allergy testing or start pulling out every delicious thing in the world from your diet. No more sugar, dairy, or wheat for you. Enjoy your brown rice and lean turkey breast. Oh dear, please don't go swimming for at least an hour after a feast like that!

Ironically, your health advocate will probably, at the same time, suggest that you do relaxing activities like meditation, deep breathing, taking warm baths, getting a massage, and hitting the sauna. These activities make you deeply relaxed, warm all over, and drowsy, just like eating a really good, complete meal that has everything your body needs will do.

You should feel a little tired after a meal—certainly more relaxed, with little desire to jump up and run. If you don't feel relaxed and a bit tired then there's something seriously wrong with your meal. It must not have enough carbs, fat, protein, salt, or calories—and your body's desire to hunt down more food stays turned on instead of powering down, feeling relaxed and ready for digestion to begin.

When we eat a good meal, insulin rises. When insulin rises, cortisol and the entire action of the sympathetic nervous system shuts down, leaving us feeling relaxed and warm and fuzzy all over. The higher your stress levels are prior to eating, the more complete that shutdown is. Thus, the longer you go without food, the more sleep-deprived you are, or the longer you've been strung out on stress hormones in a stressful situation--the bigger the post-meal coma.

The coma itself is the antidote to your stressful life. It's not an enemy, something to be avoided, or something to be lambasted by your highly caffeinated nutritionist. It's perfectly healthy, normal, natural, and in many cases quite therapeutic (just like a massage or sauna) to feel drowsy after a good meal. If you were to treat it as such and not think there is something "wrong" with it or fearfully making the assumption that the next step will be The Beetus, you could really enjoy the feeling—making lots of "ahhhhhh" and "mmmmm" sounds and grinning. I mean, what about Bob?

The point is basically that if you are experiencing a significant problem with post-meal food coma, this is either not a problem—and in fact could be a powerful form of therapy for the stress burden you are under, or it is a sign that you are overstressed somehow—most likely through lack of sleep, which I discussed earlier.

I don't have anything else definitive to say about food coma, but while we're on the topic of "hypoglycemia," I feel it is important to dispel the widely believed myth that it's bad to feel tired or sleepy after a meal. The problem isn't necessarily that you are sleepy after eating, but more likely that you are doing or not doing things that causes you to be overly sleepy after you eat (and your adrenal glands are using this as a much-needed opportunity to recharge their batteries). And the "problem," if you can even call it that (the problem is that you probably feel sleepy when your boss expects you to be focused and productive), is extremely unlikely to be attributable to true hypoglycemia.

Hyponatremia—The Other "Hypoglycemia"

Hyponatremia symptoms—from Wikipedia, the most trusted source, lol…

"Symptoms of hyponatremia include nausea and vomiting, headache, confusion, lethargy, fatigue, loss of appetite, restlessness and irritability, muscle weakness, spasms, or cramps, seizures, and decreased consciousness or coma. The presence and severity of symptoms are associated with the level of plasma sodium (salt level in the blood), with the lowest levels of plasma sodium associated with the more prominent and serious symptoms (the less the salt the more severe the symptoms). However, emerging data suggest that mild hyponatremia (plasma sodium levels at 131 mEq/ L or above) is associated with numerous complications or subtle, presently unrecognized symptoms (e.g., increased falls, altered posture and gait, reduced attention)."

Hmmm. Similar symptoms to adrenergic syndrome eh? Very similar. While it's virtually impossible to confirm this kind of thing unless you live with a nurse and have a laboratory on the premises to analyze your blood regularly, I believe that hyponatremia is a common cause of adrenergic syndrome.

Hyponatremia means low, sodium, blood. Blood is one of our extracellular (outside of the cell) fluids. A typical person has about 15 liters of extracellular fluid, and the most dominant ion in this fluid is sodium. Here are a few very interesting things to note, and why I've approached most "hypoglycemics" as "hyponatremics" with great success:

1. Those with a reduced metabolic rate have a lower threshold for water. In other words, a healthy person can drink a half liter or more of water and not have to pee for hours. When they do it is still nice and yellow in color. Those with a low metabolism; however, notoriously have water "go right through them." Even a single cup (1/4 liter) of water can induce frequent urination and adrenergic syndrome.

2. Many with a low metabolism that I have encountered have chronically low blood levels of sodium—it just seems to be a typical

manifestation of a reduced metabolic rate, and as Ray Peat claims matter-of-factly—those with a low metabolism have difficulty holding on to sodium.

3. Those who pursue healthy eating and drinking practices are typically gravitating towards foods that are very high in water content—such as fruits, vegetables, juice, raw foods, smoothies, herbal tea, and other tonics and potions. Meanwhile, they are likely to be limiting salt intake and drinking the proverbial "eight glasses of water per day." They frequently drink even more than that if they have overachiever tendencies. If water's good for ya, more must be better right?

4. Urine concentration often parallels symptoms of adrenergic syndrome, which overlap with the symptoms of hyponatremia. Taking in too much fluid causes frequent clear urination, and this is often accompanied by negative symptoms indistinguishable from "hypoglycemia."

5. In early literature on "hypoglycemia," such as Abrahamson and Pezet's 1951 classic *Body, Mind, and Sugar*, the most common aggravators of what the authors believed to be "hypoglycemia" were

beverages that are commonly consumed in excess of physiological fluid needs—soft drinks, coffee, and alcoholic beverages. They blamed the effects of the drugs and sugar content on triggering these events, but in my experience, fruit juice, caffeine-free diet drinks, and even plain old water are even bigger triggers of symptoms that could easily be perceived as "hypoglycemia." Most people I encounter have no problem with what *should* cause blood sugar crashes, but give them a watery smoothie with no salt and they may experience severe symptoms.

How many people who think they suffer from hypoglycemia actually are suffering from low salt levels? I don't know. I'd say more than 50% of cases, meaning that, in my estimation, a lot more people suffer from issues with fluid to electrolyte ratios (sodium is an electrolyte) than they do with straight blood sugar regulation problems. But it really doesn't matter. I approach both conditions similarly and neither require avoidance of carbohydrates—including pie, ice cream, cookies, and all the other pleasant things that struck fear in the heart of Abrahamson and Pezet and every nutritionist since. I believe in both cases the primary culprit is a reduced metabolic rate.

You can experiment freely for yourself using the guide coming up in the next chapter…

Self-Experimentation Guide

I have discussed many of the following things in several of my other books, including *Eat for Heat*, *Diet Recovery 2*, and most recently—*Solving the Paleo Equation*, which will actually debut *after* this book even though I wrote it several months earlier. I will try to cover the information thoroughly enough here so that if you suffer from adrenergic syndrome you will be able to get the tools you need to reduce or eliminate unpleasant symptoms. The other books are more thorough and detailed with a much greater backstory to make the recommendations seem less shocking. If you are interested, I offer my books for free on occasion so there is no extra charge, and I also offer a free 90-day Raising Metabolism eCourse on my website, which is the greatest tool I've put together to date.

You can get my free eCourse by subscribing at www.180degreehealth.com.

What are we after here? What is the goal?

I think those are very important questions for everyone to ask with any health pursuit. I like to keep things as simple and practical as possible, almost to a fault. In my experience, especially with those with adrenergic syndrome and a frequent tendency towards anxiety—the last thing on the planet you need is a list of 48 different things to think about when it comes to your diet, exercise, and lifestyle habits. Odds are that if you are like most people that read books about health, you are subtly following over 100 health tips picked up over years of health nerdism already. Let's get back to the absolute bare basics with a specific focus on the changes that sufferers of this condition have made and reaped the most reward from.

While keeping with the basics, I turn much of the focus away from the minutiae of diet, and focus on proper function. The most important functions I think you should focus on if you have hopes of truly overcoming this condition (and not just "treating it"), are:

1. Get your morning oral or rectal waking body temperature to 98 degrees F/36.7 C. Higher than that is even better, with temperatures rising

during the day to at least 98.6F/37C by late afternoon/early evening.

2. Get some nice yellow color in your urine every time you urinate, day or night, with urine frequency at once every four hours or so during the day and none at night. Also eliminate any strong, sudden urges to urinate at any time.

3. Increase your nightly sleep to eight or more hours (preferably more like nine to ten), and be able to go at least eight hours without waking up with an adrenaline surge or need to pee.

4. Keep your hands and feet warm as many hours during the day as possible. Hands and feet are usually only warm when the adrenal glands are fairly quiet. You want them to be quiet as much of the time as possible while recovering from adrenergic syndrome.

Wow. Complicated right? Seriously though, most but not all cases of adrenergic syndrome can be cleared up by achieving those four simple things. While they may seem like far-fetched goals if you haven't slept more than four hours straight in a decade or your body temperature is 94.8 degrees F, you might be surprised at how obtainable those four functional goals are. Not everyone can achieve them to perfection, to be certain. I don't want to overhype this in the slightest or sling any panaceas at you. But most, in my experience, are just a few small steps away from significantly-improved function in these four areas, and with those improvements comes anywhere from minor relief to complete obliteration of adrenergic syndrome. Let's talk about interventions you might consider in going after these improvements.

Acute Treatment

First things first. You are going to be eating carbohydrates in pursuit of improvement in the four core areas listed above. When you start eating carbohydrates, this may trigger some initial "crash" activity. Instead of trying to avoid the crash, expect it, and respond accordingly.

When you feel a crash of some kind beginning to occur—a sudden change in mood, coldness sweeping across your body, cold hands and feet, a strong urge to urinate, and other negative symptoms—eat some rapidly-absorbed carbohydrates with plenty of salt immediately. Forget about eating strict "health food" in this situation. Unrefined, whole foods digest slowly, and the longer it takes for you to take the load off of your adrenal glands, the more damage will be done. I suggest eating a good handful of something dry, refined, and instantly-absorbed into your bloodstream.

The simplest, and often most effective, is just to carry a little salt/sugar mixture with you in a little bag. The mixture should be plain old granulated white sugar mixed with a small amount of finely-ground salt. I recommend Morton's Canning and Pickling salt. I don't have a precise ratio that I recommend, but you should be able to taste the salt and it shouldn't be so salty that you find it disgusting. A big spoonful should go under or on your tongue and sit there until it dissolves into solutes that can be rapidly absorbed through the mouth's rich blood supply, going directly into your bloodstream, where it can quickly halt unpleasant crash symptoms.

Saltine crackers or pretzels are another option, and are pretty easy to carry along with you wherever you go. You shouldn't need a ton. A few should do.

If you still can't bear to eat processed food in any way, dried fruit and cheese will also work. It just takes a little longer to take effect. Whatever you choose, or whatever you are able to obtain at the time of the crash, make sure it is *concentrated*. By concentrated I mean that it is calorie-dense and not full of a bunch of water. Hence "dried fruit" instead of the recommendation for fresh fruit.

But try your best to combine sugar and salt, starch and salt, or all three. The salt is likely to be more therapeutic if you are urinating frequently during your crash, but carbohydrate is needed with the salt to have the desired effect and give quick relief of your crash symptoms. I would also take advantage of this helpful aid if you have those 2-4am wakeups with severe symptoms or difficulty falling back to sleep. It has helped many.

If all else fails, try something different! Making manipulations with your diet and lifestyle is not an exact science, but if you have a problem that you want to fix, you should be trying some new things out. The above advice *generally* works, but nothing is foolproof.

More important than the specifics of what you are eating to relieve a crash in an acute sense is that you are noticing what time of day a crash is most likely to occur. When you catch on to the trends you can start planning this snack pre-emptively—consuming it before the time of day you would expect to crash instead of waiting for the symptoms to set in. Once they've set in, it can wipe you out for days if you are particularly sensitive, so know thyself and be prepared.

But hopefully, the following interventions will give you enough "crashproofness" that the tendency to crash, and the need to rely on an acute intervention like pretzels or potato chips or sugar under your tongue, will be short-lived.

Big Breakfast

If you recall from earlier, the longer you go without food, and the higher cortisol goes, the more likely you are to have a post-meal stress event. You'll also remember that cortisol is naturally much higher in the morning for most people and that body temperature and metabolism are lower earlier in the day and higher later (with cortisol levels following that pattern). That is why people are much more likely to crash early in the day rather than late in the day (although many do crash between 8-10pm as well when aldosterone starts to reach its daily peak).

What all this points to is that breakfast is indeed a very important meal. If the vast amount of research showing breakfast's health benefits is valid, the health benefits are probably derived from a quick lowering of morning cortisol and a faster ascent to the optimal metabolic state. Overall this would lead to higher 24-hour average metabolic rate and presumably a lower total exposure to cortisol, which is arguably the most important single achievement in general health preservation. Cortisol plays a leading role in the general degenerative process seen with aging, and has close ties to almost all of the most common degenerative ailments. A great read on this, although I think they are too singularly-focused on just one of many causes of high cortisol (chronic infection), is Russ Farris and Per Marin's *The Potbelly Syndrome*.

Breakfast that is high in carbohydrates in particular, such as the classic morning cereal, seems to have even more health benefits attributed to it.

If you wish to read further evidence supporting regularly eating a high carb breakfast, here are several interesting links to government published long term statistical studies, most of which were of very large groups of male and female participants and were frequently monitored over a period of many years. The results of the studies were significant and supported the positive health benefits and also maintenance of lower body mass index (BMI), lower weight, and lowered risk of Diabetes when regularly consuming a high carbohydrate breakfast, such as ready to eat or cooked cereals. In comparison, many high protein breakfast eaters were overweight and had significantly higher BMIs and either already had, or were at greater risk for Diabetes:

http://www.ncbi.nlm.nih.gov/pubmed/16339127

http://www.ncbi.nlm.nih.gov/pubmed/18198313

http://www.ncbi.nlm.nih.gov/pubmed/14647087

http://www.ncbi.nlm.nih.gov/pubmed/12897044

http://www.ncbi.nlm.nih.gov/pubmed/16129079

http://www.ncbi.nlm.nih.gov/pubmed/21868140

http://www.ncbi.nlm.nih.gov/pubmed/19699835

http://www.ncbi.nlm.nih.gov/pubmed/18325135

http://www.ncbi.nlm.nih.gov/pubmed/18093352

But I don't care so much about statistics, theory, or having PubMed pissing contests. I'm interested more in individuals, and when helping individuals, the most important operative word is *flexibility*. With flexibility, any research, all of which eventually contradicts itself if you research any topic in great enough depth, becomes less relevant. Instead, one is free to pursue self-experimentation in a relatively free and neutral environment.

Okay, that brief primer aside, let's talk about breakfast. Like I pointed out in the chapter on hyponatremia, I find crashes due to a drop in sodium to fluid ratios in the body are as prevalent, probably more prevalent, than genuine blood sugar problems. In the morning when metabolic rate is reduced, the body is much more sensitive to sudden changes in fluid levels. And what are most people doing? Waking up to a big glass of water or mega coffee is very common, and if there is any food involved it's usually something extremely watery with very little salt. Smoothies are perhaps the worst. Big glasses of juice and watery breakfast cereal isn't much help either—unless they are well-balanced with foods with a lower water content and plenty of salt.

What I would do if I were you is keep the big focus on carbohydrates in the morning as is customary in most cultures, but instead choose less watery foods and ramp up the salt. The goals are to feel warm after breakfast, not have a big adrenaline surge, keep those hands and feet toasty, and keep that urine from getting clear. For many with a real problem in the metabolism department, this can seem like an impossibility at first. But it's not. You'll get there little buckaroo. Keep at it.

If you notice that your tendency to crash is greatest between breakfast and lunch and you are generally colder in the morning than the afternoon and evening, I would also recommend that you "frontload" your calories towards the first half of the day. By frontloading I mean eating most of your food by about 1-2pm. If you eat 3,000 calories per day, that might mean a breakfast of 1,000 calories, a 400-calorie snack, and a 1,200-calorie lunch. By that time you'll be stuffed and a light dinner of a baked potato, a salad, or some soup will suffice.

This food, until you get your metabolism really high and no longer have post-meal crashes, should be very calorie-dense and palatable. Someone in great metabolic shape can eat a fruit salad with a cup of coffee for breakfast and feel fine. Those with adrenergic syndrome almost always fare better on foods like pancakes with tons of maple syrup, salty fried potatoes, eggs with lots of cheese and salt, French toast, and other classics (like leftover pizza!)—and only enough fluids to satisfy thirst, but no more.

Water with lemon, fresh juice, big ice-cold smoothies, oatmeal cooked in water with no salt added, big hunks of melon—in my experience these watery foods are kryptonite to a person with a low metabolism. You may be able to consume those later in the day and feel fine, but you'll probably need some very calorie-dense foods in the morning, and calorie-dense foods are almost always the ones no one considers to be "healthy." Your biofeedback will likely tell you otherwise. Be open-minded as you find what food or combinations of foods "gets you hot" so-to-speak.

If you crash right after a big breakfast like this anyway, eat again. Nibble your way through the entire morning if you have to, but keep chowing down until you get warm! Once you get nice and warm, you're likely to have a much better day. There's also no need to stuff your face when you are already nice and toasty. When you're warm, eat all the damn health food you want—if you have any appetite left.

The main thing when trying to overcome a crash tendency at a certain time of day is that you are trying to eat more calories, carbohydrates, and salt *in proportion to total fluids*. The body fluids have a ratio of sodium to water. You want to make sure that the net sum of food, salt, and fluids equals a concentrated "soup" that is going to build up the strength of your body fluids, not dilute it at its most vulnerable point in the day.

Hopefully that's enough talk about breakfast. I do believe that the pro-metabolic, anti-stress effects of food are one of the primary weapons against adrenergic syndrome. Let's talk about one more food-related thing and then move on. There is more to proper function than food, and I'm sick of everybody obsessively talking about it—especially me.

Night Eating

If you are a late-evening (after 8pm) crasher or a 2-4am crasher, adjusting food and fluids in the evening can have just as powerful of an effect as what was covered in the breakfast discussion. The same general rule applies—eating heavier, richer, more calorie-dense foods with lots of carbs and salt at the time of day you tend to crash makes sense and usually works.

For after-dinner crashes you might eat a dessert and something salty before bed. I usually recommend eating whatever it takes to avoid having to go to bed with cold toes. Most of my followers with this problem report potato chips and ice cream to be the most magical combination, but you need to experiment and find what works and what you like. For every person that gets sweaty-hot after ice cream there is a person who gets ice cold for hours after eating it.

Even more screwy is the 2-4am crash. Usually the best approach is to follow metabolism-stimulating guidelines in general, as this problem at the root seems to mostly be caused by the surge in adrenaline that happens when metabolic energy starts to sputter at the daily body temperature low point.

But night eating occasionally is of pivotal importance. There is no foolproof way to guide you here, but know that this nighttime crash can be worsened by eating light at night and in general, or it can be caused by eating too heavy. Strange I know, but it's true.

When you go experimenting with it for yourself, it should be pretty clear what group you fall into. Eat very light after about 2pm, strongly frontloading your calorie intake as described earlier. Do this for several days to a week consistently. If you feel like death and your sleep has steadily worsened over the course of that week, that's probably not the right daily food structure for you. If, however, you notice almost instant relief from longstanding sleep problems when eating very lightly from lunch onward, stick with it.

I'd say a good third of bad sleep problems that I've encountered can be tremendously improved by adjusting food intake later in the day—calories up or down. Another third can be tremendously improved with a basic pro-metabolism approach. Body temperature up, sleep improved. That leaves a remaining third with no sleep improvement, but being able to fix so many sleep problems with such simple and easy interventions is a really cool thing. You're welcome world.

Overall Calorie Intake

Son of a...!!! I really thought that was going to be the last of the food talk. One more thing!

I'm not an advocate of counting calories in a general sense. It's imprecise at best and far too neurotic for most people. Life was carried out quite successfully for a couple billion years before the word "calorie" was even created. If you have a low body temperature and aren't seeing any improvement at all, it might be time to see how much you're eating. It's physiologically impossible to raise your metabolic rate while eating an insufficient amount of food. To fuel metabolic rate you must eat enough food. In the modern era there are a lot of people that are chronically undereating, and they are just the type of person that would purchase a book like this.

There is no precise way to predict how many calories a person needs to maintain a high metabolic rate, as there are so many variables—the greatest of which is how many pounds of lean tissue you carry around on your body and how much you move around. But a general calculation I use to *estimate* caloric needs for optimal metabolic performance is…

Males: Lean bodyweight in pounds X 20

Females: Lean bodyweight in pounds X 18

Lean bodyweight is basically how much you would weigh if you were lean enough to see some pretty good muscle definition in your whole body.

Metabolism goes through an unavoidable slowdown as we age due to the natural wear and tear on our mitochondria—the power plants of metabolism on the cellular level. If you are over the age of 30, multiply the figures from above by 100 minus the number of years over 30 you are divided by 100.

Okay, that was confusing. If you are 50, you are 20 years past 30. 100-20 = 80. 80 divided by 100 is 0.8. Multiply the calorie counts above for your gender by 0.8.

So a 50 year-old lady with a lean weight of 120 pounds would be:

120 X 18 = 2,160

2160 X 0.8 = 1,728

Those calculated calorie counts are for general maintenance of a high metabolic rate, and that's if you aren't doing much intentional exercise. You may be able to get by with slightly less, but odds are if your metabolism comes up significantly you will start spontaneously moving around more and burning more calories—thus needing even more. Also, if your metabolism is very low, you may need an even bigger surplus to trigger an actual increase in metabolic rate back to normal. I've used even higher figures in my book *Diet Recovery 2*, for example.

That's all I wanted to say about calorie tracking. Make sure you're eating enough or you'll never make progress.

Relaxing Activities

The goal is to raise metabolic rate and stifle the stress response from being overactive in adrenergic syndrome. Why limit oneself to only dietary interventions? While ample amounts of food is a necessary prerequisite to proper metabolic function, it's just one tool.

I highly recommend taking relaxing activities very seriously. Especially like those enjoyable activities listed below that are known to put the mind into an alpha brain wave state or lower. Relaxation can be quite powerful at dictating the physiological state your body retreats to.

Adrenal hormones tend to ramp up mental energy and increase the frequency of brain waves. That's why they give hardcore stimulants to those with attention problems. That's also why people drink coffee to shed the brain fog and feel more alert. While I love those beta brain waves—I'm producing plenty right now—interventions designed to slow brain wave activity allow the physical body to follow suit and begin to relax.

Here are some common ways to unwind and veg out, in turn smoothing over a crash or preventing them in a general sense. None of these are rocket science or anything new, but many have been shamefully ignored or forgotten about by those in search of more exotic "cures." There's beauty in the basics. Make some of the following things a ritual, and you may find the therapeutic effects to greatly exceed your expectations:

1. Warm baths, Jacuzzi, or saunas
2. Lying flat on your back and closing your eyes
3. Going outdoors in a quiet place
4. Meditating or other techniques for quieting the conscious mind (such as hypnosis)
5. Exercise (in some cases, for some this is more stressful than it is de-stressing)
6. Massage

7. Listening to relaxing and inspiring music

There are countless other ways to relax. Do whatever you find to have a soothing effect for you, but really try to prioritize this kind of thing and work it into your daily rituals.

Sleep

This is a huge one. Sleep, for me personally, is my master. The quality and quantity of my sleep is by far the greatest determinant of my overall health and well-being. I wish I liked to do it more! I'm naturally pretty upbeat and creative with a constant stream of ideas flowing through my hyperactive mind. Sleep never sounds like a fun thing to do. I'm almost never in the mood for it. The only time I ever get a lot of sleep is when I'm out camping. It's dark and cold and there's nothing to do!
I think that's part of the problem. Our modern environment is great in so many ways. My curiosity never ends, and I never want to turn away entertainment either. I mean, is there really a time when I'm NOT in the mood to watch an 80's movie? No. Never. In fact, in the last 24 hours I've watched *Funny Farm, Baby Boom,* and *When Harry Met Sally*. No joke. And I don't see myself getting sick of those movies any time soon. It's been a quarter century, and they are still just as enjoyable now as they were the first time I watched them. *When Harry Met Sally* is even better.

Of course, not everyone is capable of sleeping well. I understand that. Some people have physiological stress that is simply overbearing—making deep, uninterrupted sleep an impossibility that the methods discussed in this book can't fully address. Hopefully some of the interventions I mentioned earlier will assist you with that if you find getting adequate sleep impossible even when you make the time.

For the rest of us, please get more sleep. I know it's boring, but the decreasing length of the average night's sleep is what I consider to be the most alarming health trend of the 20th century, trumping even the significance of the industrial pollutants, processed food, and crippling sedentarism that have become a way of life. Without modern gadgets and glowing boxes, how much do I sleep? At least 11 hours a night. It is the most incredible-feeling thing ever.

As boring and disheartening as it may be to hear of sleep's importance, I can almost guarantee that a biologically-normal amount of sleep (almost all creatures sleep WAY more than humans) will improve your adrenergic syndrome. The research results on sleep's positive effects on leptin, metabolic rate, glucose metabolism, cortisol, and more is unanimously good.

Minerals

Minerals are heavily involved with blood sugar regulation and other key biological processes. While I have very little experience with using mineral supplements in a precise way to improve adrenergic syndrome, a practitioner that I enlist a tremendous amount of trust is Dr. Garrett Smith. We have even co-authored a book together.

In 2013 Dr. Smith has been performing hair mineral analysis on his patients. In the context of "eating for heat" so-to-speak in line with some of the above recommendations, he's reported excellent results, including full resolution of his own post-breakfast crash tendency. I always trust the reports of actual clinicians above theorists, especially when that clinician is so knowledgeable about the real fundamentals of proper function.

I make absolutely no money whatsoever from my endorsement of hair mineral analysis or of Dr. Garrett Smith. Nor is it a favor to him. It is a favor to you, especially if you have followed some of the basics in this chapter to a dead end. You can contact Dr. Smith about getting tested and rebalancing your body's mineral reserves (which involves supplementation primarily with minerals) by sending his office manager an email: adminNMSA@gmail.com

Other Supplements

I rarely advise a person to seek outside supplementation, primarily because most people need to hear a much stronger message about adhering to some of the basic fundamentals of health rather than the pill, powder, and potion approach to health. However, there comes a time and place when basic dietary and lifestyle design has been exhausted and been found to come up short. At that point it's reasonable to pursue supplementation, most notably the primary pro-metabolism hormones such as progesterone and thyroid hormone (T3 or desiccated thyroid). Occasionally I hear reports of large doses of iodine working fairly well, too.

I cannot guide you in any way on dosage or specific recommendations, but seeking out some help in this department from a licensed professional may be just the breakthrough you needed. Just don't jump too quickly to reach for a pill when you haven't at least attempted to resolve the issue through your own personal health practices.

Exercise

It's rare in modern society for a person to be truly overexerting themselves and causing themselves problems from it. However, overexertion isn't all that rare amongst people that read health books, and the threshold for exercise is quite low when you aren't eating and sleeping well, which most health-conscious people aren't in my experience. Really, only lemonade for ten days? Good luck with that.

If your body temperature is reduced and you struggle to get it to rise to the targets mentioned earlier—and you are a fitness fanatic—you might consider taking it easy for a while and slowly reintroducing exercise in quantities and intensities that don't suppress your body temperature or worsen your adrenergic syndrome.

Conclusion

I'm not one for elaborate conclusions. I think the book has been pretty simple and straightforward. The main takeaways are:

1. Symptoms that most people call "hypoglycemia" aren't caused by having blood sugar levels fall below normal.

2. The symptoms associated with hypoglycemia are triggered by stress at the root.

3. Physiological stress hormone levels tend to become elevated more easily when metabolic rate is low due to many factors.

4. The old-school recommendation to eat frequent meals high in protein and low in carbohydrates is unnecessary, potentially harmful, and doesn't address the root problem.

5. Many cases of supposed "hypoglycemia" are actually hyponatremia—or low salt levels proportional to the water content in our extracellular fluids.

6. By focusing on some fundamentals of good function such as proper body temperature, urine concentration and frequency, body warmth, and sleep—and seeking improvement in those areas, most cases of adrenergic syndrome can be resolved or at the very least improved.

7. Interventions that raise metabolic rate and lower exposure to stress such as eating more salt, sugar, and starch and more calorie-dense food in general when body temperature is at its low point, getting more sleep, and spending more time engaged in relaxing activities like meditation and warm baths are simple but powerful.

8. Minerals and supplementation with thyroid hormone and others can provide additional therapy where some of the recommendations fail.

9. If none of that works, try something else.

10. Matt Stone is the man

That's all I was trying to get across—particular emphasis on #10.

I hope this information serves you well. If this book brings up additional questions that you need answered, please ask them! I am not unapproachable in the slightest. The easiest way to get in touch with me is to subscribe to the mailing list on my website, which includes a 90-day series of email-delivered "lessons" on raising metabolic rate. You can actually reply to those emails with your questions and comments, and I'll be more than happy to answer them.

Best of luck to you in all of your health adventures.

Sincerely,
Matt Stone
www.180degreehealth.com

Raising Metabolism eCourse

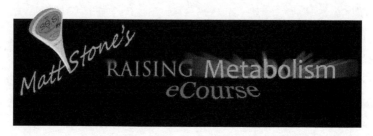

In nearly a decade of intensive research, I've been led to believe that metabolic rate is by far the most important health marker to focus on. You can get all of my latest research and precise tactics on raising metabolic rate in my exhaustive 90-day Raising Metabolism eCourse, available for FREE when you subscribe at www.180degreehealth.com

Excerpt from *Solving the Paleo Equation*

Types of Stressors

As Selye claims, stress can be produced by virtually any agent. So the following list is by no means exhaustive. No list could ever comprehensively encompass the myriad things that elicit a stress response. Below are some of the major ones, as well as the most common, especially among the health-conscious. We'll call these the Dirty Dozen (and hopefully that won't cause any cliché stress).

1. **Psychological stress** This is obviously the biggest and the baddest of the stressors; it also comes in the greatest variety. Psychological stress is particularly powerful because our psyche has a very strong impact on our physiology. It can also stick

around, sometimes for years, and become chronic and debilitating, unlike the acute yet relatively insignificant stress of, say, some granny driving like Stevie Wonder, her car swerving in slow motion toward your Mini Cooper (the most common source of acute stress in the state of Florida). A painful event from even decades ago can still affect your body, especially if you frequently revisit the experience in your mind. Psychological stress comes in the form of holding grudges, anxiety, divorce, being overly stressed about work, relationship dissatisfaction, doing a job you hate, financial stress, babies crying in the night, dealing with the tragic loss of life of those close to you, social anxiety, body image insecurity—the list goes on and on. If a memory or thought can trigger a strong emotion any time you think about it, it's probably a great source of stress.

2. **Diet stress** Most of you probably wouldn't consider dieting as a source of stress, yet for some it's the mother of all stressors. Chronic calorie deprivation and carbohydrate restriction are the most extreme dietary stressors, and they are stressors that no amount of meditation or spiritual awakening can overcome. There are other diet stressors, like restricting a food that you wish you could eat— denying your cravings can be a huge stress. Likewise, continually gorging on a food that you don't tolerate well can create an inflammatory

reaction and is also a source of dietary stress. Binge eating in response to your self-imposed dietary restrictions is another stress, often topped with guilt that lasts well beyond the physical distress. Eating, in general, is one of the primary de-stressing activities, so you have to account for not only causing stress but also missing out on one of your primary stress relievers.

3. **Inflammation stress** There is a massive amount of research on the huge role that inflammation plays in most diseases. Well, guess what? Stress heightens inflammation and inflammation heightens stress. And there is no doubt that anything that sets off inflammation will also initiate a release of inflammatory mediators like cortisol, which is the body's main stress hormone. Ever take hydrocortisone or prednisone for a nasty allergic reaction? These are pharmaceutical variations of our own cortisol and provide an anti-inflammatory effect. But keep in mind that chronic inflammation can lead to chronic hypercortisolism—too much cortisol. Chronic infections, of which there are endless varieties (including the many familiar viral and bacterial infections as well as common things like gum disease or dental infection), can trigger this high inflammation, chronic high-stress situation. There is also very strong evidence that modern human cells are primed for producing overzealous immune and inflammatory responses in general—

hence the epidemics of food allergies, asthma, auto-immune disease, and other hyperinflammatory conditions. Much more on this to come in Part Two: Nutrition because much of this type of inflammation can be improved with simple dietary changes.

4. **Sleep stress** Some research suggests that the average night's sleep a century ago was around nine hours. Today we average closer to seven hours, and many people get far less. Chronic sleep deprivation is certainly known to be a major source of chronic stress, and, like harsh dietary restriction, this is particularly detrimental because not only are you causing stress by missing out on sleep, you are missing out on a primary antistress tool. It's a double whammy. (Yes, I just said *double whammy*. I try to say it any chance I get.)

5. **Medication stress** There are many medications that can cause chronic stress on several fronts, due to their active ingredients and their actions. Even some antidepressants (Prozac and friends) are known to raise cortisol levels. There are also many habit-forming substances, such as alcohol and nicotine, that may lower cortisol in the short term but over time lead to a higher overall stress burden. Prescription, over-the-counter, and recreational stimulants—from Adderall to Sudafed to weight loss pills to your morning coffee—are being used in greater and greater amounts world- wide. Stimulants

are yet another way of digging your spurs into your stress system.

6. **Exercise stress** Exercise is a form of stress. There's no question about that. In the right amounts and in the right context (when you are eating lots of food, carbs in particular; you're getting good sleep; and you have low to moderate stress levels), exercise is one of the highly beneficial stresses. But, as Garrett will get into in greater detail, there is no question that exercise can also turn sour. And that's because fewer and fewer people in this day and age (and fewer still among those with a health and fitness fetish) are exercising in the right quantity, dosage, and context. While exercise has undeniably wonderful attributes in a general sense, for many individuals it is one of the greatest, if not *the* greatest, sources of stress.

7. **Light stress** There's no doubt that one of the most "un-Paleo" things we do in the modern world is totally mess around with normal and natural light exposure. Bright light raises cortisol. This may sound like a bad thing, but a peak in cortisol in the morning hours when the sun is bright and shining is normal and healthy.

In the modern world, however, we have managed to extend the number of hours we're exposed to bright light with our shiny new gadgets. We now keep ourselves awake, bright lights a-blazin' and cortisol a-soarin', in a "wired" state after dark. I'm talking primarily about those glowing, luminous boxes like computer screens and televisions. At best, we miss out on much-needed sleep and have trouble naturally winding down—which is stressful. At worst, this late-night light can increase total stress hormone exposure. There's no doubt that higher cortisol levels in general increase the risk for developing many health problems, such as the constellation of factors that comprise metabolic syndrome (insulin resistance, high blood pressure, high blood glucose, abdominal fat storage, etc.). There is also evidence that constantly being bathed in electromagnetic frequencies (EMF) from all the electrical gadgets and appliances that surround us takes a toll, increasing stress. While it is definitely *not* our intention to make you paranoid enough to retreat into the wilderness stark-naked and barefoot to avoid the ravages of modernity, going to bed closer to sunset, sleeping in as dark a room as possible, and, at the very least, dimming your computer monitor after dark are all fairly practical interventions that are powerful stress reducers.

8. **Seasonal stress** Winter in and of itself is a stressor, and the human body simply doesn't function at its peak mentally, emotionally, or physically during cold, dark winters. While I don't necessarily encourage you to move to the tropics to avoid this, it's certainly good to become aware of seasonal stress and adjust your diet, exercise, and

lifestyle patterns accordingly. It may be customary in January to starve oneself and jump on a big, unsustainable exercise kick to burn off holiday excesses, but it is definitely an example of poor timing.

9. **Sexual stress** While this could be filed under the broader category of psychological stress, there are some physical considerations to take into account as well. Not getting enough sex is very stressful, but so is getting too much. In a world full of constant sexual bombardment through television, advertisements, and, of course, pornography, many people—men especially—put themselves under great stress by engaging in excessive sex and masturbation. This may sound ridiculous, but sex uses a lot of reserve energy, and it can get drained, just like anything else. In addition, too much stress crushes sex drive and function.

10. **Irregularity stress** One thing overlooked in today's chaotic world is the importance of regular rhythms and patterns. There is even some evidence that having a consistent meal schedule rather than an erratic one promotes a healthy metabolic rate, cholesterol levels, and more. In real-world practice, the simple act of having a regular and consistent schedule for exercise, meals, bedtime, and waking time can be very helpful in stress management. As Scott Abel, one of the fitness industry's leading experts, says, "The body thrives on regularity."

Anytime there is chaos instead of consistency, our bodies are much quicker to dive into a stressful alarm state.

11. **Noise stress** Loud and obnoxious noise is another often-overlooked stressor. If it has the power to annoy, you can be sure it's a trigger of the stress response. Construction workers who fail to use ear protection at noisy job sites experience dramatic rises in cortisol. While you may have little control over your exposure to noise in your own life, it is still a potent source of stress for some. The good news is that most can become desensitized to noise over time and have a minimal physical reaction to it.

12. **Stress-list stress** Reading long lists of things that can trigger stress triggers stress. Before, you were unaware of how harmful stress is and the many ways it is entering your life. Now, you are deathly afraid of developing "the Beetus" and having your leg amputated a couple decades from now because you own a television, winter is approaching, and you have a toothache. You are staying up even later now researching diabetes prevention on the Internet and scouring late-night infomercials for magic cures. While this rant is obviously going above and beyond the call of duty to lighten things up a little bit, it is a good lesson to learn in general. Don't read too much about all the harmful things in our world, in our diets, and in

everything that is more or less normal these days. Being weird and isolated from everyone in a state of health paranoia is a huge stress, too. You might consider backing off your fierce health and nutrition research habit. Ignorance is sometimes bliss in this regard. If you are going to read health stuff, dim the screen on your e-book reader or laptop when you do it. You know, light stress and all. And as Kent was instructed by God in the movie *Real Genius,* "Stop playing with yourself!"

Now you can identify a few of the more prevalent kinds of stress. In the next chapter we'll get into something even more useful: how to assess your overall stress burden through common indicators

About the Author

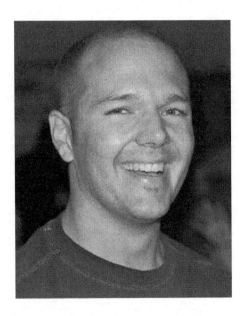

Matt Stone is the founder of 180DegreeHealth. He is an independent health researcher and bestselling author of more than 15 books, including *Eat for Heat*, a #1 Amazon bestselling book since its debut in December, 2012. Most of his research has drawn him towards metabolic rate and how many basic functions (digestion, reproduction, aging, immunity, inflammation, mood, circulation, sleep) perform better when metabolic rate is optimized. He is most notable for his criticisms of extreme diets and exposing many false diet industry claims, as well as his works on raising metabolic rate through simple changes in diet and lifestyle. You can keep up with Matt's at http://www.180degreehealth.com and reading his many books available only at Amazon.

Made in the USA
San Bernardino, CA
11 July 2016